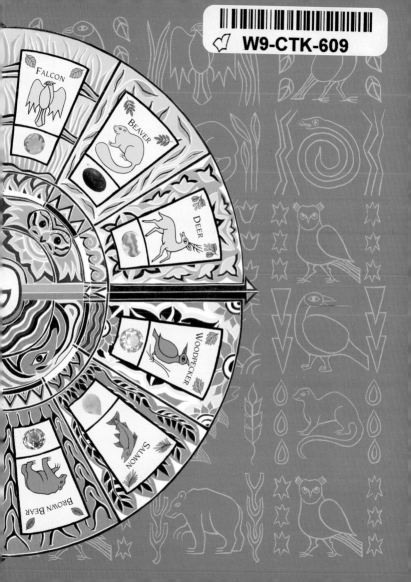

FALCON

BEAVER

DEER

WOODPECKER

SALMON

BROWN BEAR

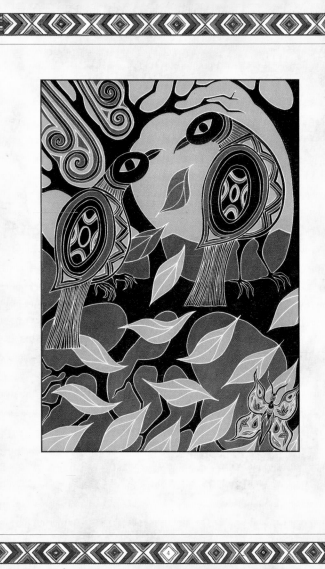

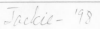
Jackie - '93

THE LITTLE LIBRARY OF EARTH MEDICINE

CROW

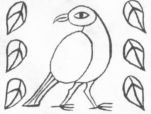

Kenneth Meadows

Illustrations by Jo Donegan

DORLING KINDERSLEY
LONDON • NEW YORK • SYDNEY • MOSCOW

A DORLING KINDERSLEY BOOK

Managing editor: Jonathan Metcalf
Managing art editor: Peter Cross
Production manager: Michelle Thomas

The Little Library of Earth Medicine was
produced, edited and designed by
GLS Editorial and Design
Garden Studios, 11-15 Betterton Street
London WC2H 9BP

GLS Editorial and Design
Editorial director: Jane Laing
Design director: Ruth Shane
Project designer: Luke Herriott
Editors: Claire Calman, Terry Burrows, Victoria Sorzano

Additional illustrations: Roy Flooks 16, 17, 31; John Lawrence 38
Special photography: Mark Hamilton
Picture credits: American Natural History Museum 8-9, 12, 14-15, 32

First published in Great Britain in 1998
by Dorling Kindersley Limited
9 Henrietta Street, London WC2E 8PS

2 4 6 8 10 9 7 5 3 1

A CIP catalogue record for this book is available from the British Library

UK ISBN 0 7513 0520 0   AUSTRALIAN ISBN 1 86466 037 6

Reproduced by Kestrel Digital Colour Ltd, Chelmsford, Essex
Printed and bound in Hong Kong by Imago

CONTENTS

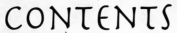

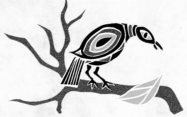

INTRODUCING
EARTH MEDICINE

To Native Americans, medicine is not an external
substance but an inner power that is found in
both Nature and ourselves.

Earth Medicine is a unique method of personality profiling that draws on Native American understanding of the Universe, and on the principles embodied in sacred Medicine Wheels.

Native Americans believed that spirit, although invisible, permeated Nature, so that everything in Nature was sacred. Animals were perceived as acting as

Shaman's rattle
Shamans used rattles to connect with their inner spirit. This is a Tlingit shaman's wooden rattle.

messengers of spirit. They also appeared in waking dreams to impart power known as "medicine". The recipients of such dreams honoured the animal species that appeared to them by rendering their images on ceremonial and everyday artefacts.

NATURE WITHIN SELF
Native American shamans – tribal wisemen – recognized similarities between the natural forces prevalent during the seasons and the characteristics of those born

*"Spirit has provided you with an opportunity to
study in Nature's university."* Stoney teaching

during corresponding times of the year. They also noted how personality is affected by the four phases of the Moon – at birth and throughout life – and by the continual alternation of energy flow, from active to passive. This view is encapsulated in Earth Medicine, which helps you to recognize how the dynamics of Nature function within you and how the potential strengths you were born with can be developed.

Animal ornament
To the Anasazi, who carved this ornament from jet, the frog symbolized adaptability.

MEDICINE WHEELS
Native American cultural traditions embrace a variety of circular symbolic images and objects. These sacred hoops have become known as Medicine

Wheels, due to their similarity to the spoked wheels of the wagons that carried settlers into the heartlands of once-Native American territory. Each Medicine Wheel showed how different objects or qualities related to one another within the context of a greater whole, and how different forces and energies moved within it.

One Medicine Wheel might be regarded as the master wheel because it indicated balance within Nature and the most effective way of achieving harmony with the Universe and ourselves. It is upon this master Medicine Wheel (see pp.10–11) that Earth Medicine is structured.

Feast dish
Stylized bear carvings adorn this Tlingit feast dish. To the American Indian, the bear symbolizes strength and self-sufficiency.

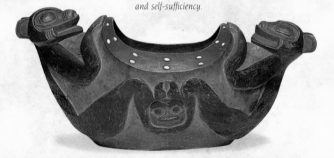

THE MEDICINE WHEEL

The outer Wheel is divided into twelve birth times, each of which has its own animal totem, and stone, tree, and colour affinities.

At the hub of the Wheel, surrounded by representations of Elements, Directions, and energy flow, is the Wakan-Tanka – symbol of invisible energies coming into physical reality.

Season of birth
Each of the twelve segments relates to a specific time of year (see pp.12–13).

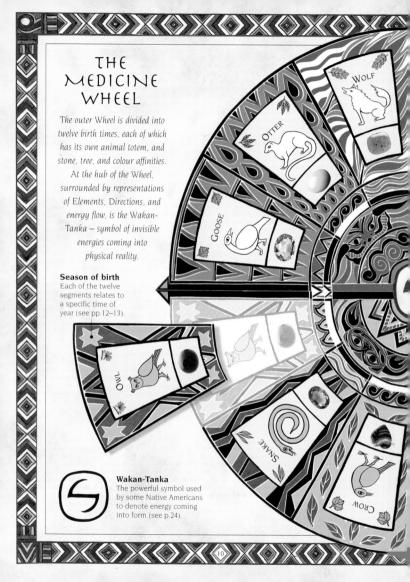

WOLF

OTTER

GOOSE

OWL

SNAKE

CROW

Wakan-Tanka
The powerful symbol used by some Native Americans to denote energy coming into form (see p.24).

10

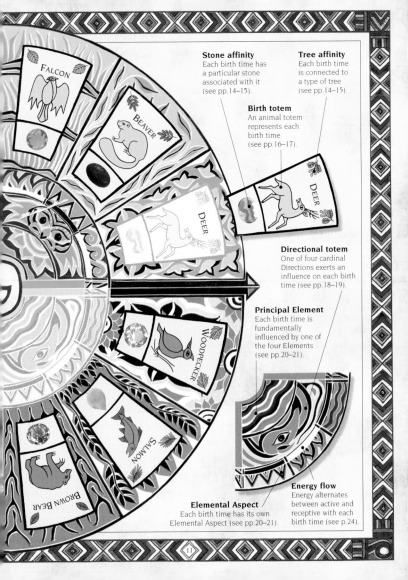

Stone affinity
Each birth time has a particular stone associated with it (see pp.14–15).

Tree affinity
Each birth time is connected to a type of tree (see pp.14–15).

Birth totem
An animal totem represents each birth time (see pp.16–17).

Directional totem
One of four cardinal Directions exerts an influence on each birth time (see pp.18–19).

Principal Element
Each birth time is fundamentally influenced by one of the four Elements (see pp.20–21).

Energy flow
Energy alternates between active and receptive with each birth time (see p.24).

Elemental Aspect
Each birth time has its own Elemental Aspect (see pp.20–21).

FALCON

BEAVER

DEER

DEER

WOODPECKER

SALMON

BROWN BEAR

THE TWELVE
BIRTH TIMES

THE STRUCTURE OF THE MEDICINE WHEEL IS BASED
UPON THE SEASONS TO REFLECT THE POWERFUL
INFLUENCE OF NATURE ON HUMAN PERSONALITY.

T he Medicine Wheel classifies human nature into twelve personality types, each corresponding to the characteristics of Nature at a particular time of the year. It is designed to act as a kind of map to help you discover your strengths and weaknesses, your inner drives and instinctive behaviours, and your true potential.

The four seasons form the basis of the Wheel's structure, with the Summer and Winter solstices and the Spring and Autumn equinoxes marking each season's passing. In Earth Medicine,

each season is a metaphor for a stage of human growth and development. Spring is likened to infancy and the newness of life; and Summer to the exuberance of youth and of rapid development. Autumn represents the fulfilment that mature adulthood brings, while Winter symbolizes the accumulated wisdom that can be drawn upon in later life.

Each seasonal quarter of the Wheel is further divided into three periods, making twelve time segments altogether. The time of your birth determines the direction from which

Seasonal rites
*Performers at the Iroquois mid-
Winter ceremony wore masks made
of braided maize husks. They danced
to attune themselves to energies that
would ensure a good harvest.*

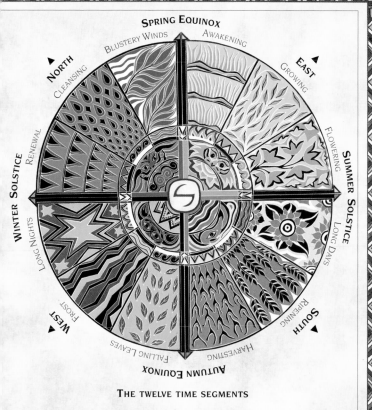

The twelve time segments within the wheel, reading around:

SPRING EQUINOX

BLUSTERY WINDS — AWAKENING

NORTH — CLEANSING — GROWING — EAST

RENEWAL — FLOWERING

WINTER SOLSTICE — SUMMER SOLSTICE

LONG NIGHTS — LONG DAYS

WEST — FROST — RIPENING — SOUTH

FALLING LEAVES — HARVESTING

AUTUMN EQUINOX

THE TWELVE TIME SEGMENTS

you perceive life, and the qualities imbued in Nature in that season are reflected in your core character.

Each of the twelve time segments, or birth times, is named after a feature in the natural yearly cycle. For

example, the period after the Spring equinox is called Awakening time because it is the time of new growth, while the segment after the Autumn equinox is named after the falling leaves that characterize that time.

THE SIGNIFICANCE OF
TOTEMS

NATIVE AMERICANS BELIEVED THAT TOTEMS – ANIMAL SYMBOLS – REPRESENTED ESSENTIAL TRUTHS AND ACTED AS CONNECTIONS TO NATURAL POWERS.

A totem is an animal or natural object adopted as an emblem to typify certain distinctive qualities. Native Americans regarded animals, whose behaviour is predictable, as particularly useful guides to categorizing human patterns of behaviour.

A totem mirrors aspects of your nature and unlocks the intuitive knowledge that lies beyond the reasoning capacity of the intellect. It may take the form of a carving or moulding, a pictorial image, or a token of fur, feather, bone, tooth, or claw. Its presence serves as an immediate link with the energies it represents. A totem is therefore more effective than a glyph or symbol as an aid to comprehending non-physical powers and formative forces.

PRIMARY TOTEMS

In Earth Medicine you have three primary totems: a birth totem, a Directional totem, and an Elemental totem. Your *birth totem* is the embodiment of core characteristics that correspond with the dominant aspects of Nature during your birth time.

Symbol of strength

The handle of this Tlingit knife is carved with a raven and a bear head, symbols of insight and inner strength.

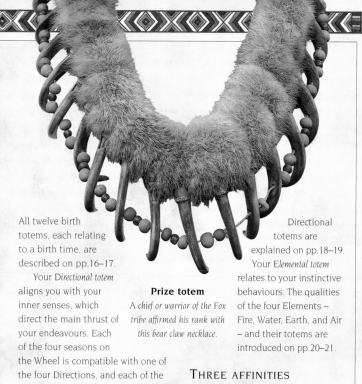

All twelve birth totems, each relating to a birth time, are described on pp.16–17.

Your *Directional totem* aligns you with your inner senses, which direct the main thrust of your endeavours. Each of the four seasons on the Wheel is compatible with one of the four Directions, and each of the Directions is represented by a totem. For example, Spring is associated with the East, where the sun rises, and signifies seeing things in new ways; its totem is the Eagle. The four

Prize totem

A chief or warrior of the Fox tribe affirmed his rank with this bear claw necklace.

Directional totems are explained on pp.18–19.

Your *Elemental totem* relates to your instinctive behaviours. The qualities of the four Elements – Fire, Water, Earth, and Air – and their totems are introduced on pp.20–21.

THREE AFFINITIES

Each birth time also has an affinity with a tree, a stone, and a colour (see pp.36–41). These three affinities have qualities that can strengthen you during challenging times.

"If a man is to succeed, he must be governed not by his inclination, but by an understanding of the ways of animals..." Teton Sioux teaching

THE TWELVE
BIRTH TOTEMS

THE TWELVE BIRTH TIMES ARE REPRESENTED BY TOTEMS,
EACH ONE AN ANIMAL THAT BEST EXPRESSES THE
QUALITIES INHERENT IN THAT BIRTH TIME.

Earth Medicine associates an animal totem with each birth time (the two sets of dates below reflect the difference in season between the northern and southern hemispheres). These animals help to connect you to the powers and abilities that they represent. For an in-depth study of the Crow birth totem, see pp.28–29.

FALCON
21 March–19 April (N. Hem)
22 Sept–22 Oct (S. Hem)
Falcons are full of initiative, but often rush in to make decisions they may later regret. Lively and extroverted, they have enthusiasm for new experiences but can sometimes lack persistence.

DEER
21 May–20 June (N. Hem)
23 Nov–21 Dec (S. Hem)
Deer are willing to sacrifice the old for the new. They loathe routine, thriving on variety and challenges. They have a wild side, often leaping from one situation or relationship into another without reflection.

BEAVER
20 April–20 May (N. Hem)
23 Oct–22 Nov (S. Hem)
Practical and steady, Beavers have a capacity for perseverance. Good homemakers, they are warm and affectionate but need harmony and peace to avoid becoming irritable. They have a keen aesthetic sense.

WOODPECKER
21 June–21 July (N. Hem)
22 Dec–19 Jan (S. Hem)
Emotional and sensitive, Woodpeckers are warm to those closest to them, and willing to sacrifice their needs for those of their loved ones. They have lively imaginations but can be worriers.

SALMON
22 July–21 August (N. Hem)
20 Jan–18 Feb (S. Hem)

Enthusiastic and self-confident, Salmon people enjoy running things. They are uncompromising and forceful, and can occasionally seem a little arrogant or self-important. They are easily hurt by neglect.

OWL
23 Nov–21 Dec (N. Hem)
21 May–20 June (S. Hem)

Owls need freedom of expression. They are lively, self-reliant, and have an eye for detail. Inquisitive and adaptable, they have a tendency to overextend themselves. Owls are often physically courageous.

BROWN BEAR
22 August–21 Sept (N. Hem)
19 Feb–20 March (S. Hem)

Brown Bears are hardworking, practical, and self-reliant. They do not like change, preferring to stick to what is familiar. They have a flair for fixing things, are good-natured, and make good friends.

GOOSE
22 Dec–19 Jan (N. Hem)
21 June–21 July (S. Hem)

Goose people are far-sighted idealists who are willing to explore the unknown. They approach life with enthusiasm, determined to fulfil their dreams. They are perfectionists, and can appear unduly serious.

CROW
22 Sept–22 Oct (N. Hem)
21 March–19 April (S. Hem)

Crows dislike solitude and feel most comfortable in company. Although usually pleasant and good-natured, they can be strongly influenced by negative atmospheres, becoming gloomy and prickly.

OTTER
20 Jan–18 Feb (N. Hem)
22 July–21 August (S. Hem)

Otters are friendly, lively, and perceptive. They feel inhibited by too many rules and regulations, which often makes them appear eccentric. They like cleanliness and order, and have original minds.

SNAKE
23 Oct–22 Nov (N. Hem)
20 April–20 May (S. Hem)

Snakes are secretive and mysterious, hiding their feelings beneath a cool exterior. Adaptable, determined, and imaginative, they are capable of bouncing back from tough situations encountered in life.

WOLF
19 Feb–20 March (N. Hem)
22 August–21 Sept (S. Hem)

Wolves are sensitive, artistic, and intuitive – people to whom others turn for help. They value freedom and their own space, and are easily affected by others. They are philosophical, trusting, and genuine.

THE INFLUENCE OF THE
DIRECTIONS

ALSO KNOWN BY NATIVE AMERICANS AS THE FOUR
WINDS, THE INFLUENCE OF THE FOUR DIRECTIONS IS
EXPERIENCED THROUGH YOUR INNER SENSES.

Regarded as the "keepers" or "caretakers" of the Universe, the four Directions or alignments were also referred to by Native Americans as the four Winds because their presence was felt rather than seen.

DIRECTIONAL TOTEMS
In Earth Medicine, each Direction or Wind is associated with a season and a time of day. Thus the Autumn birth times – Falling Leaves time, Frost time, and Long Nights time –

all fall within the West Direction, and evening. The Direction to which your birth time belongs influences the nature of your inner senses.

The East Direction is associated with illumination. Its totem is the Eagle – a bird that soars close to the Sun and can see clearly from height. The South is the Direction of Summer and the afternoon. It signifies growth and fruition, fluidity, and emotions. Its totem, the Mouse, symbolizes productivity, feelings, and an ability to perceive detail.

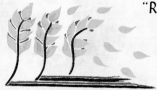

"Remember...the circle of the sky, the stars, the super-natural Winds breathing night and day...the four Directions." Pawnee teaching

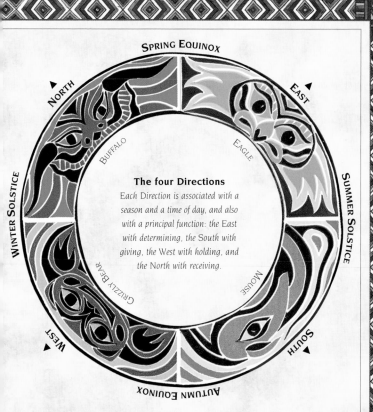

SPRING EQUINOX

NORTH

EAST

WINTER SOLSTICE

SUMMER SOLSTICE

BUFFALO

EAGLE

The four Directions

Each Direction is associated with a season and a time of day, and also with a principal function: the East with determining, the South with giving, the West with holding, and the North with receiving.

GRIZZLY BEAR

MOUSE

WEST

SOUTH

AUTUMN EQUINOX

The West is the Direction of Autumn and the evening. It signifies transformation – from day to night, from Summer to Winter – and the qualities of introspection and conservation. Its totem is the Grizzly Bear, which represents strength

drawn from within. The North is the Direction of Winter and the night, and is associated with the mind and its sustenance – knowledge. Its totem is the Buffalo, an animal that was honoured by Native Americans as the great material "provider".

THE INFLUENCE OF THE ELEMENTS

THE FOUR ELEMENTS – AIR, FIRE, WATER, AND EARTH –
PERVADE EVERYTHING AND INDICATE THE NATURE OF
MOVEMENT AND THE ESSENCE OF WHO YOU ARE.

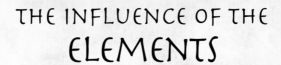

Elements are intangible qualities that describe the essential state or character of all things. In Earth Medicine, the four Elements are allied with four fundamental modes of activity and are associated with different aspects of the self. Air expresses free movement in all directions; it is related to the mind and to thinking. Fire indicates expansive motion; it is linked with the spirit and with intuition. Water signifies fluidity; it

Elemental profile
*The configuration of
Crow is Air of Earth.
Earth is the Principal
Element and Air the
Elemental Aspect.*

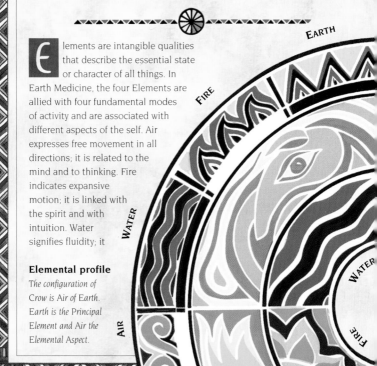

EARTH

FIRE

WATER

AIR

WATER

FIRE

has associations with the soul and the emotions. Earth symbolizes stability; it is related to the physical body and the sensations.

ELEMENTAL DISTRIBUTION

On the Medicine Wheel one Element is associated with each of the four Directions – Fire in the East, Earth in the West, Air in the North, and Water in the South. These are known as the Principal Elements.

AIR

WATER

EARTH

AIR

FIRE

EARTH

The four Elements also have an individual association with each of the twelve birth times – known as the Elemental Aspects. They follow a cyclical sequence around the Wheel based on the action of the Sun (Fire) on the Earth, producing atmosphere (Air) and condensation (Water).

The three birth times that share an Elemental Aspect belong to the same Elemental family or "clan", with a totem that gives insight into its key characteristics. Crow people belong to the Butterfly clan (see pp.34–35).

ELEMENTAL EMPHASIS

For each birth time, the qualities of the Elemental Aspect usually predominate over those of the Principal Element, although both are present to give a specific configuration, such as Fire of Earth (for Crow's, see pp.34–35). For Falcon, Woodpecker, and Otter, the Principal Element and the Elemental Aspect are identical (for example, Air of Air), so people of these totems tend to express that Element intensely.

THE INFLUENCE OF THE
MOON

THE WAXING AND WANING OF THE MOON DURING ITS
FOUR PHASES HAS A CRUCIAL INFLUENCE ON THE
FORMATION OF PERSONALITY AND HUMAN ENDEAVOUR.

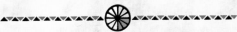

Native Americans regarded the Sun and Moon as indicators respectively of the active and receptive energies inherent in Nature (see p.24), as well as the measurers of time. They associated solar influences with conscious activity and the exercise of reason and the will, and lunar influences with subconscious activity and the emotional and intuitive aspects of human nature.

The Waxing Moon

This phase lasts for approximately eleven days. It is a time of growth and therefore ideal for developing new ideas and concentrating your efforts into new projects.

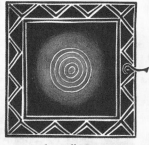

The Full Moon

Lasting about three days, this is when lunar power is at its height. It is therefore a good time for completing what was developed during the Waxing Moon.

THE FOUR PHASES

There are four phases in the twenty-nine-day lunar cycle, each one an expression of energy reflecting a particular mode of activity. They can be likened to the phases of growth of a flowering plant through the seasons: the emergence of buds (Waxing Moon), the bursting of flowers (Full Moon), the falling away of flowers (Waning Moon), and the germination of seeds (Dark Moon). The influence of each phase can be felt in two ways: in the formation of personality and in day-to-day life.

The energy expressed by the phase of the Moon at the time of your birth has a strong influence on personality. For instance, someone born during the Dark Moon is likely to be inward-looking, whilst a person born during the Full Moon may be more expressive. Someone born during a Waxing Moon is likely to have an outgoing nature, whilst a person born during a Waning Moon may be reserved. Consult a set of Moon tables to discover the phase the Moon was in on *your* birthday.

In your day-to-day life, the benefits of coming into harmony with the Moon's energies are considerable. Experience the energy of the four phases by consciously working with them. A Native American approach is described below.

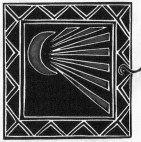

The Waning Moon
A time for making changes, this phase lasts for an average of eleven days. Use it to improve and modify, and to dispose of what is no longer needed or wanted.

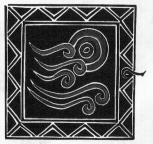

The Dark Moon
The Moon disappears from the sky for around four days. This is a time for contemplation of what has been achieved, and for germinating the seeds for the new.

THE INFLUENCE OF
ENERGY FLOW

THE MEDICINE WHEEL REFLECTS THE PERFECT BALANCE OF THE COMPLEMENTARY ACTIVE AND RECEPTIVE ENERGIES THAT CO-EXIST IN NATURE.

Energy flows through Nature in two complementary ways, which can be expressed in terms of active and receptive, or male and female. The active energy principle is linked with the Elements of Fire and Air, and the receptive principle with Water and Earth.

Each of the twelve birth times has an active or receptive energy related to its Elemental Aspect. Travelling around the Wheel, the two energies alternate with each birth time, resulting in an equal balance of active and receptive energies, as in Nature.

Active energy is associated with the Sun and conscious activity. Those whose birth times take this principle prefer to pursue experience. They are conceptual, energetic, outgoing, practical, and analytical. Receptive energy is associated with the Moon and subconscious activity. Those whose birth times take this principle prefer to attract experience. They are intuitive, reflective, conserving, emotional, and nurturing.

THE WAKAN-TANKA

At the heart of the Wheel lies an S-shape within a circle, the symbol of the life-giving source of everything that comes into physical existence – seemingly out of nothing. Named by the Plains Indians as Wakan-Tanka (Great Power), it can also be perceived as energy coming into form and form reverting to energy in the unending continuity of life.

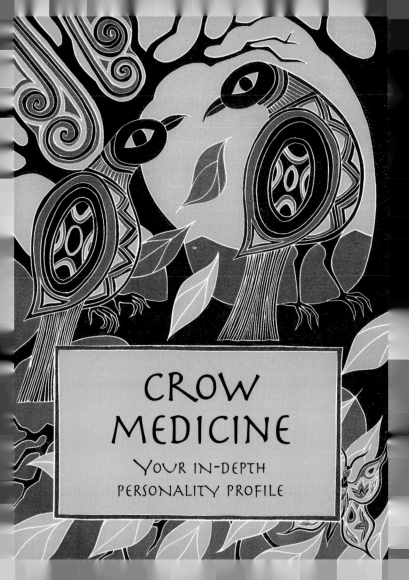

CROW MEDICINE

YOUR IN-DEPTH PERSONALITY PROFILE

FALLING LEAVES TIME

THE REFLECTIVE NATURE OF AUTUMN BEGINS IN THE FIRST BIRTH TIME OF THE SEASON, LENDING THOSE BORN THEN THE QUALITIES OF INTROSPECTION AND BALANCE.

Falling Leaves time is one of the twelve birth times, the fundamental division of the year into twelve seasonal segments (see pp.12–13). As the first period of the Autumn cycle, it is the time of year when the Sun's energy wanes as Nature prepares for its period of dormancy. Trees shed their leaves and animals increase their food stores in preparation for Winter.

INFLUENCE OF NATURE

The qualities and characteristics imbued in Nature at this time form the basis of your own nature. So, just as all living creatures are building up their resources in readiness for the barren months ahead, so, if you were born during Falling Leaves time, you have an introspective, resourceful nature, and you require regular periods of rest to recharge your batteries. At this time of year the number of daylight hours falls to equal the number of hours of darkness. This balance in Nature is reflected in your own equitable nature, which enables you to see the good and bad in situations, and to enjoy creating harmony between people.

This is a time of thanksgiving for all that Nature has provided during the Spring and Summer months, and the beginning of a more contemplative, introspective period. In a similar way, you appreciate the qualities of others, and are thoughtful and considerate in your approach to people and situations.

STAGE OF LIFE

This time of year might be compared to the middle years of life. In human development terms, it is a period of consolidation, when the knowledge gained and the skills developed during the first half of your life are appraised. It is a time of contemplation and evaluation of all that you have achieved so far in life, and of the development of greater self-reliance and inner strength.

ACHIEVE YOUR POTENTIAL

Your desire for balance and justice means you have a strong need to justify your actions. It also means that you like to share your good fortunes with others and that you thrive only in a harmonious atmosphere.

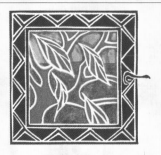

Nature's energy
Nature begins its dormant phase in this, the first cycle of Autumn after the Autumn equinox. Trees start to shed their leaves, animals seek out their winter homes and store up food for the barren months ahead.

Your appreciation of all points of view and all kinds of people makes you a highly popular friend and a sociable creature. At work you excel when operating as part of a team and you make an excellent negotiator. However, when playing a diplomatic role, try not to allow your desire for harmony and fairness over-ride your sense of justice or loyalty to your ideals. Draw on your inner resources to cultivate your capacity for persistence and tenacity.

"Life is a circle from childhood to childhood; so it is with everything where power moves." Black Elk teaching

BIRTH TOTEM
THE CROW

THE ESSENTIAL NATURE AND CHARACTERISTIC
BEHAVIOUR OF THE CROW EXPRESSES THE PERSONALITY
TYPE OF THOSE BORN DURING FALLING LEAVES TIME.

Like the crow, people born during Falling Leaves time are adaptable, sociable, and loyal. If you were born at this time, you have a fair-minded, discreet, and considerate nature that thrives in an orderly and friendly environment.

Easy-going and diplomatic, you enjoy the company of others and prefer working as part of a team rather than on your own. A model of discretion, you can be trusted to keep a confidence, and make a loyal and popular friend and colleague. Your thoughtful approach to people and situations enables you to appreciate every side of any argument and to perceive all the options available at any time.

However, your desire to maintain harmony and to be fair in your dealings with others often makes you indecisive and over-cautious. Such hesitancy sometimes results in missed opportunities, and can perplex friends and colleagues. Ensure that more of your dreams are fulfilled by worrying less about pleasing others or making mistakes.

Crow power

Sociable, lively, and adaptable, the crow also expresses the co-operative and gregarious aspects of the friendly, talkative people born at this time.

HEALTH MATTERS

Usually cheerful, contented, and even-tempered, you can easily become depressed, sullen, and quarrelsome when surrounded by confusion, disorder, or unpleasant behaviour. At such times, you may find that you suffer muscular problems in the abdomen and lower back. Remove yourself from the situation to relax and recharge your batteries. Also, avoid over-indulging in food and drink as you tend to be prone to digestive disorders.

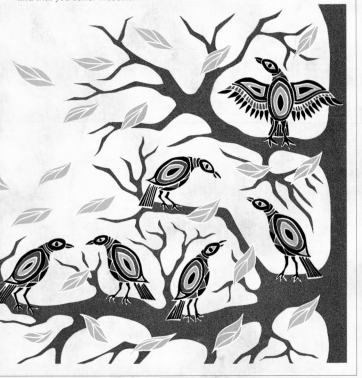

THE CROW AND
RELATIONSHIPS

CHEERFUL AND GREGARIOUS, CROW PEOPLE ARE
USUALLY POPULAR. THEY MAKE ROMANTIC AND
ADAPTABLE PARTNERS BUT MAY PROVE FICKLE IN LOVE.

O utgoing, sociable creatures, Crow people, like their totem animal, crave the company of others. If your birth totem is Crow, you are at your best in a group, so usually enjoy being with friends or working as part of a team. Your desire for harmony makes you a skilful diplomat, soothing discord and creating a positive atmosphere. However, your adaptable nature can make you compromise your integrity and individuality in your wish to avoid conflict.

LOVING RELATIONSHIPS
Romantic Crows are in love with love but may find the imperfect nature of real relationships a disappointment. Flirtatious male Crow is charming and considerate but fickle, while female Crow is seductive without letting her

heart rule her head. Both tend to have a high sex drive.

When problems in relationships arise, it is sometimes because of your periodic moodiness, when you can be stubborn or morose. You also find it difficult to take responsibility for yourself, which can create an imbalance in your relationships.

COPING WITH CROW
Crow people are charming, adaptable, and tolerant so they are usually good company. Be clear and keep to the point when dealing with them because they dislike confusion. They are attuned to atmosphere, and may become sullen and irritable in adverse situations. You can trust Crows to be loyal and discreet, but beware of mistaking their friendliness or flirtatiousness for affection.

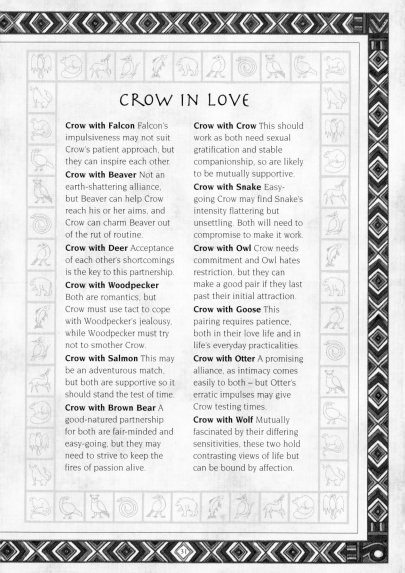

CROW IN LOVE

Crow with Falcon Falcon's impulsiveness may not suit Crow's patient approach, but they can inspire each other.

Crow with Beaver Not an earth-shattering alliance, but Beaver can help Crow reach his or her aims, and Crow can charm Beaver out of the rut of routine.

Crow with Deer Acceptance of each other's shortcomings is the key to this partnership.

Crow with Woodpecker Both are romantics, but Crow must use tact to cope with Woodpecker's jealousy, while Woodpecker must try not to smother Crow.

Crow with Salmon This may be an adventurous match, but both are supportive so it should stand the test of time.

Crow with Brown Bear A good-natured partnership for both are fair-minded and easy-going, but they may need to strive to keep the fires of passion alive.

Crow with Crow This should work as both need sexual gratification and stable companionship, so are likely to be mutually supportive.

Crow with Snake Easy-going Crow may find Snake's intensity flattering but unsettling. Both will need to compromise to make it work.

Crow with Owl Crow needs commitment and Owl hates restriction, but they can make a good pair if they last past their initial attraction.

Crow with Goose This pairing requires patience, both in their love life and in life's everyday practicalities.

Crow with Otter A promising alliance, as intimacy comes easily to both – but Otter's erratic impulses may give Crow testing times.

Crow with Wolf Mutually fascinated by their differing sensitivities, these two hold contrasting views of life but can be bound by affection.

DIRECTIONAL TOTEM
THE GRIZZLY BEAR

THE GRIZZLY BEAR SYMBOLIZES THE INFLUENCE OF
THE WEST ON CROW PEOPLE, WHO CAN BETTER FIND
DIRECTION IN LIFE BY LOOKING INWARD FOR GUIDANCE.

F alling Leaves time, Frost time, and Long Nights time all fall within the quarter of the Medicine Wheel associated with the West Direction or Wind.

Grizzly bear bowl
This Tlingit wooden bowl is carved in the shape of a bear, which is associated with inner strength.

The West is aligned with Autumn and dusk, and it is associated with introspection, consolidation, maturity, and the wisdom that stems from experience. The power of the West's influence is primarily with the physical, and its principal function is the power of holding. It takes as its totem the self-sufficient grizzly bear.

The specific influence of the West on Crow people is on clarity of purpose, enabling you to find a stronger sense of direction in life and the right outlet for your talents. It is also associated with the qualities of adaptability and the power to impart knowledge.

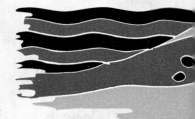

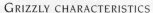

GRIZZLY CHARACTERISTICS

In Autumn, the powerful grizzly bear makes careful preparation for hibernation, storing up its inner strength for reawakening in Spring. Hence, Native Americans associated it with resourcefulness and self-reliance. It was seen as introspective because it seemed to be thoughtful about its actions; as a totem, it encourages you to look within for guidance and to learn from the past to bring wisdom to your decisions.

If your Directional totem is Grizzly Bear, you are likely to have a capacity for endurance, the resolve to face up to your weaknesses, and the courage to learn from experience.

The spirit of the West

The Sun sets in the West, symbolizing reflection; the Grizzly Bear totem signifies self-reliance.

ELEMENTAL TOTEM
THE BUTTERFLY

LIKE THE BUTTERFLY, WHICH FLITS FROM PLACE TO
PLACE, CROW PEOPLE'S RESTLESS TEMPERAMENT
REQUIRES VARIETY AND ROOM TO MANOEUVRE.

The Elemental Aspect of Crow people is Air. They share this Aspect with Deer and Otter people, who all therefore belong to the same Elemental family or "clan" (see pp.20–21 for an introduction to the influence of the Elements).

THE BUTTERFLY CLAN

Each Elemental clan has a totem to provide insight into its essential characteristics. The totem of the Elemental clan of Air is Butterfly, which symbolizes a quick, lively, restless, and changeable nature.

The butterfly flits here and there, seeking variety, and settling only where the atmosphere is harmonious.

Free to change

The butterfly symbolizes the fundamental quality of the Element of Air: free movement.

So if you belong to this clan you will have a lively personality and be constantly on the move – physically, mentally, and emotionally.

Quick-witted, thoughtful, and imaginative, you are full of ideas, which you are keen to communicate to others. You dislike being restricted either physically or mentally. You are quick and impatient, and crave stimulation and plenty of opportunity to express yourself.

ELEMENTAL PROFILE

For Crow people, the predominant Elemental Aspect of changeable Air is fundamentally affected by the qualities of your Principal Element – persistent Earth. Consequently, if you were born at this time you are likely to have an abundance of energy together with a dependable, tenacious nature, enabling you to press on towards your goals in spite of difficulties and disappointments.

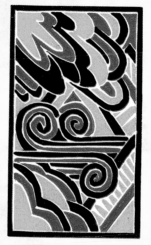

Air of Earth
The Element of Air feeds Earth, generating expansiveness and dependability.

You may seem indecisive, driven by the urge to change that is inherent in Air and the desire for stability that is inherent in Earth. Sometimes your love of harmony and capacity to remain neutral makes you slow to realize your own needs – which can lead to feelings of frustration or resentment.

At times like these, or when you are feeling low or lacking in energy, try the following revitalizing exercise. Find a quiet spot outside, away from the polluting effects of traffic and the activities of others, and, for several minutes, breathe slowly and deeply.

With each in-breath, acknowledge that you are drawing into yourself the energizing power of the life-force, which is being absorbed by every cell of your being, revitalizing and refreshing your whole body.

STONE AFFINITY
AZURITE

BY USING THE GEMSTONE WITH WHICH YOUR OWN
ESSENCE RESONATES, YOU CAN TAP INTO THE POWER OF
THE EARTH ITSELF AND AWAKEN YOUR INNER STRENGTHS.

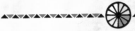

Gemstones are minerals that are formed within the Earth itself in an exceedingly slow but continuous process. Native Americans valued gemstones not only for their beauty but also for being literally part of the Earth, and therefore possessing part of its life-force. They regarded gemstones as being "alive" – channellers of energy that could be used in many ways: to heal, to protect, or for meditation.

Every gemstone has a different energy or vibration. On the Medicine Wheel, a stone is associated with each birth time, the energy of which resonates with the essence of those

Polished azurite

Azurite, here banded with malachite, has a gentle vibration that is thought to improve self-confidence.

born during that time. Because of this energy affiliation, your gemstone can be used to help bring you into harmony with the Earth and to create balance within yourself. It can enhance and develop your good qualities and endow you with the qualities or abilities you need.

ENERGY RESONANCE

Crow people have an affinity with azurite – a copper mineral with an opaque blue colour, often intergrown with malachite. Azurite contains imperfections that actually enhance its beauty – an inspiration for Crow people, who need to realize that

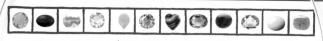

ACTIVATE YOUR GEMSTONE

Obtain a piece of azurite and cleanse it by holding it under cold running water. Let it dry naturally, then, holding the stone with both hands, raise it to your mouth and blow on it sharply and hard three or four times to impregnate it with your breath. Next, hold it firmly and silently welcome it into your life as a friend and helper. When you are feeling unclear or are facing a dilemma, use the azurite to help you meditate on the issue. Find a quiet spot to sit without fear of interruption and take the azurite in your right hand – your "activity" hand. Focus on the problem and allow your affinity stone to bring you clarity. Listen for the still, small voice of your inner self.

there can be value and potential even in something flawed. Native Americans regarded azurite as sacred, believing it helped people to become attuned to their nobler aspects and to express them in everyday life. They also used it as a detoxifying elixir and to release blocked energy.

If your birth totem is Crow, you may find azurite helpful in expanding your awareness, especially about

Azurite power

To benefit most from its effect, wear or carry a piece of azurite. If worn as a ring, it should be on the right hand, which is the hand of activity.

yourself. It enhances clarity and insight, making it a valuable aid when your urge to keep the peace means you lose sight of your principles. Keeping a piece of azurite also helps you to eliminate indecision, often a problem for you.

"The outline of the stone is round; the power of the stone is endless." Lakota Sioux teaching

TREE AFFINITY
VINE

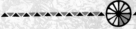

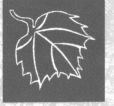

Trees have an important part to play in the protection of Nature's mechanisms and in the maintenance of the Earth's atmospheric balance, which is essential for the survival of the human race.

Native Americans referred to trees as "Standing People" because they stand firm, obtaining strength from their connection with the Earth. They therefore teach us the importance of being grounded, whilst at the same time listening to, and reaching for, our higher aspirations. When

respected as living beings, trees can provide insight into the workings of Nature and our own inner selves.

On the Medicine Wheel, each birth time is associated with a particular kind of tree, the basic qualities of which complement the nature of those born during that time. Crow people have an affinity with the vine. A vigorous climber, the vine flourishes when grown over a support. Like Crow people, it excels when in partnership. Wine, made from the vine's grapes, adds life to many a

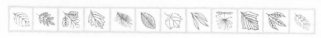

CONNECT WITH YOUR TREE

Appreciate the beauty of your affinity tree and study its nature carefully, for it has an affinity with your own nature.

The vine is a vigorous, woody-stemmed, deciduous climber which thrives in a warm climate. When grown over a support, its large, beautiful leaves provide welcome shade. Different types yield grapes either for eating or for wine-making.

Try the following exercise when you need to revitalize your inner strength. Stand beside your affinity tree. Place the palms of your hands on the plant or gently but firmly hold a leaf in each hand. Inhale slowly and experience energy from the tree's roots flow through your body. If easily available, obtain a cutting or twig from your affinity tree to keep as a totem or helper.

social occasion, easing tension like the popular and sociable Crow. In times of friction, misunderstandings, and potential discord, Crow people can tap into their own powers to promote harmony by connecting with their tree (see panel above).

PERSISTENT AMBITION

If your birth totem is Crow, you are idealistic and resourceful, but you also have a tendency to frivolity and indecision which can limit the extent of your achievements and leave you feeling underfulfilled. At times, your real need for harmony can lead you to make uneasy compromises.

Just as the vine overcomes awkward obstacles to advance and grow, so you can find the power to persist and succeed. Call on the vine's help, drawing on its quality of tenacity; it will help you renew your inner strength and nurture your own capacity to be persistent in the pursuit of your goals and dreams.

"All healing plants are given by Wakan-Tanka; therefore they are holy." Lakota Sioux teaching

COLOUR AFFINITY
BLUE

Enhance your positive qualities by using the power of your affinity colour to affect your emotional and mental states.

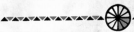

Each birth time has an affinity with a particular colour. This is the colour that resonates best with the energies of the people born during that time. Exposure to your affinity colour will help to encourage a positive emotional and mental response, while exposure to colours that clash with your affinity colour will have a negative effect on your sense of well-being.

Blue resonates with Crow people. A primary colour, uninfluenced by other colours, blue is associated with spirituality and intuitive wisdom. It is a calm, quiet, non-intrusive colour that embodies introspection, harmony, and a strong sense of

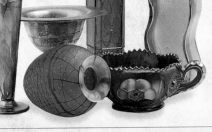

Colour scheme
Let a blue colour theme be the thread that runs through your home, from the ornaments and table settings to the fixtures and fittings, walls and floors.

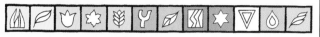

BREATHE IN YOUR COLOUR

Take a small solid object that is entirely blue, such as a stone, a paperweight, an ornament, or an item of craftwork. Place it near an open window where it can be seen and stand before it with your legs slightly apart, so that your weight is evenly distributed.

Focus on the colour and inhale slowly through the nose. Imagine that the air you breathe in is the colour of the object. Hold the breath for a few seconds and feel that colour filtering through your entire body, energizing every cell. Breathe out slowly. Pause, then begin the sequence again. Continue this rhythmic colour breathing for three or four minutes to experience the full positive effects.

duty. Blue is a colour of tranquillity and freedom of movement and ideas. It suggests integrity, sincerity, openness, idealism, co-operation with others, compassion, and devotion to higher aspirations.

COLOUR BENEFITS

Strengthen your aura and enhance your positive qualities by introducing shades of blue to the interior decor of your home. Spots of colour can make all the difference. A blue-tinted lampshade, or a decorative blue bowl or vase, for example, can alter the ambience of a room, or try covering the floor with a blue-patterned rug or the sofa with cushions that feature blue.

If you need a confidence boost, wear something that contains blue. Whenever your energies are low, practise the colour breathing exercise outlined above to balance your emotions, awaken your creativity, and help you to feel joyful.

"The power of the spirit should be honoured with its colour." Lakota Sioux teaching

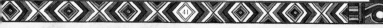

WORKING THE WHEEL
LIFE PATH

CONSIDER YOUR BIRTH PROFILE AS A STARTING POINT IN
THE DEVELOPMENT OF YOUR CHARACTER AND THE
ACHIEVEMENT OF PERSONAL FULFILMENT.

each of the twelve birth times is associated with a particular path of learning, or with a collection of lessons to be learned through life. By following your path of learning you will develop strengths in place of weaknesses, achieve a greater sense of harmony with the world, and discover inner peace.

YOUR PATH OF LEARNING
For Crow people, the first lesson on your path of learning is to cultivate a

sense of your own individuality and independence. Your sociable and easy-going nature, together with your ability to appreciate all points of view, means that you sometimes find it difficult to maintain a sense of your own identity and that your own needs become submerged under the needs of others. Try not to allow your desire for harmony and the pleasure you take in belonging and

"Each man's road is shown to him within his own heart. There he sees all the truths of life." Cheyenne teaching

sharing compromise your integrity: do not allow yourself to become all things to all men.

Crow people also need to overcome hesitancy and indecisiveness. Because of your innate sense of fairness and ability to see every aspect of a situation or argument, you find it difficult to decide in favour of one particular line of action or one individual over another. Next time you have to make a decision limit the amount of time you spend weighing up the issues and then act according to your convictions.

Your third lesson is to establish a more principled attitude to life. By acting with integrity you will win the respect of others and increase your self-esteem. By increasing your self-confidence you will be less likely to subscribe to the mentality of the group and avoid difficult decisions, and more likely to take full responsibility for your life.

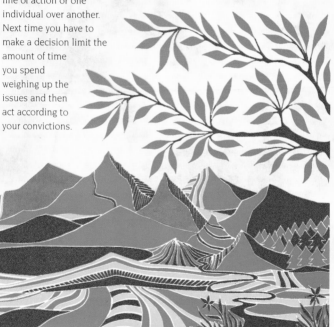

WORKING THE WHEEL
MEDICINE POWER

HARNESS THE POWERS OF OTHER BIRTH TIMES TO
TRANSFORM YOUR WEAKNESSES INTO STRENGTHS AND
MEET THE CHALLENGES IN YOUR LIFE.

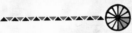

The whole spectrum of human qualities and abilities is represented on the Medicine Wheel. The totems and affinities associated with each birth time indicate the basic qualities with which those born at that time are equipped.

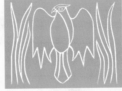

Complementary affinity

A key strength of Falcon – weak in Crow – is the ability to act with determination.

Study your path of learning (see pp.42–43) to identify those aspects of your personality that may need to be strengthened, then look at other birth times to discover the totems and affinities that can assist you in this task. For example, your Elemental profile is Air of Earth (see pp.34–35), so for balance you need the adaptive nature of Water and the enthusiasm of Fire. Woodpecker's Elemental profile is Water of Water and Salmon's is Fire of Water, so meditate on these birth totems. In addition, you may find it useful to study the profiles of the other two members of your Elemental clan of Butterfly – Deer and Otter – to discover how the same Elemental Aspect can be expressed differently.

Also helpful is the birth totem that sits opposite yours on the Medicine Wheel, which contains qualities that complement or enhance your own. This is known as your complementary affinity, which for Crow people is Falcon.

ESSENTIAL STRENGTHS

D escribed below are the essential strengths of each birth totem. To develop a
quality that is weak in yourself or that you need to meet a particular
challenge, meditate upon the birth totem that contains the attribute you need.
Obtain a representation of the relevant totem – a claw, tooth, or feather; a
picture, ring, or model. Affirm that the power it represents is within you.

Falcon medicine is the power of
keen observation and the ability to
act decisively and energetically
whenever action is required.

Beaver medicine is the ability to
think creatively and laterally – to
develop alternative ways of doing or
thinking about things.

Deer medicine is characterized by
sensitivity to the intentions of others
and to that which might be
detrimental to your well-being.

Woodpecker medicine is the ability
to establish a steady rhythm
throughout life and to be tenacious in
protecting all that you hold dear.

Salmon medicine is the strength to
be determined and courageous in the
choice of goals you want to achieve
and to have enough stamina to see a
task through to the end.

Brown Bear medicine is the ability
to be resourceful, hardworking, and
dependable in times of need, and to
draw on inner strength.

Crow medicine is the ability to
transform negative or non-productive
situations into positive ones and to
transcend limitations.

Snake medicine is the talent to
adapt easily to changes in
circumstances and to manage
transitional phases well.

Owl medicine is the power to see
clearly during times of uncertainty
and to conduct life consistently,
according to long-term plans.

Goose medicine is the courage to do
whatever might be necessary to
protect your ideals and adhere to
your principles in life.

Otter medicine is the ability to
connect with your inner child, to be
innovative and idealistic, and to
thoroughly enjoy the ordinary tasks
and routines of everyday life.

Wolf medicine is the courage to act
according to your intuition and
instincts rather than your intellect,
and to be compassionate.

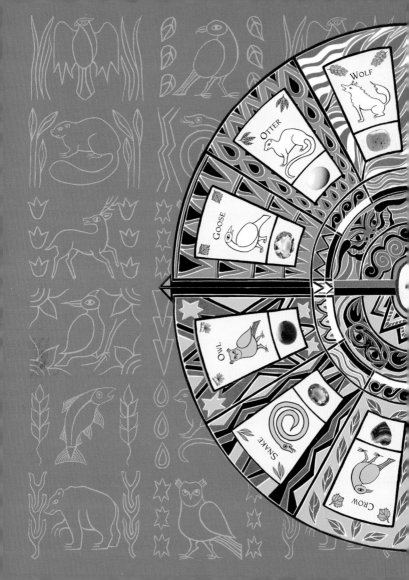